WILDERNESS SELF RELIANCE

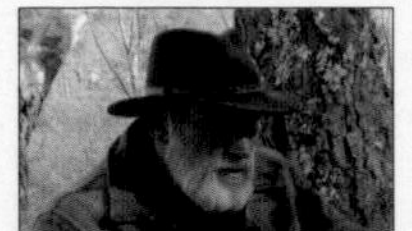

My Pathfinder Outdoor Survival Guides offer you the most simple and common sense approach to being prepared for a survival situation. If you practice the skills and techniques that are discussed in these guides, you will be in a far superior position when the situation arises.

Most important is that you develop the ability to adapt, improvise and overcome adversity by learning to use what is available to you. And that you stay firm in your belief that you CAN survive – never give up.

The Pathfinder School System®

Created as a teaching tool for my students in Wilderness Self Reliance, the Pathfinder School System represents the wisdom of the ancient scouts who ventured ahead of nomadic tribes to find fresh areas to support their community.

These "Pathfinders" had to accurately identify the perfect spot to sustain their tribes – they had to recognize the resources that would afford food, shelter, water, medicines and protection – the very same resources a person would need today. This system is designed to introduce you to the knowledge you will need to increase your survivability.

A simple survival kit is something to have in your pack or vehicle to help you survive any emergency situation. The contents will help you secure warmth, shelter, water and a method to signal for help.

Before You Go

Plan – Be sure someone knows where you are going, when you should return, and have a commitment from them to establish search & rescue if you don't report on time. Make this a habit – we don't plan to get lost, however once you are lost, it is too late to plan.

Be knowledgeable – Study your environment. Your ability to find water, build a shelter, make fire and find food will be greatly enhanced by a familiarity with terrain, vegetation and climate.

Be equipped – Build and practice the use of your survival kit components. The kit contents that I advocate save you the most exertion and make the most difference to your survivability. **Don't just buy them – practice using them.** Master their use before you head into the wilderness.

Dave Canterbury is a master woodsman with over 20 years of experience working in many dangerous environments. He has taught survival and survival methods to hundreds of students and professionals in the US and around the world. His common sense approach to survivability is recognized as one of the most effective systems of teaching known today. For information on Pathfinder programs and materials visit http://www.thepathfinderschoolllc.com.

N.B. – The publisher makes no representation or warranties with respect to the accuracy, completeness, correctness or usefulness of this information and specifically disclaims any implied warranties of fitness for a particular purpose. The advice, strategies and/or techniques contained herein may not be suitable for all individuals. The publisher shall not be responsible for any physical harm (up to and including death), loss of profit or other commercial damage. The publisher assumes no liability brought or instituted by individuals or organizations arising out of or relating in any way to the application and/or use of the information, advice and strategies contained herein.

Waterford Press publishes reference guides that introduce readers to nature observation, outdoor recreation and survival skills. Product information is featured on the website: **www.waterfordpress.com**

Text & illustrations © 2012, 2023 Waterford Press Inc. All rights reserved. Images marked IC © Iris Canterbury 2012, 2023. Cover photo © Shutterstock. To order or for information on custom published products please call 800-434-2555 or emailorderdesk@waterfordpress.com. For permissions or to share comments emaileditor@waterfordpress.com. 2306502

$7.95 U.S.
$ 9.95 CAN

ISBN 978-1-58355-705-1
50795
9 781583 557051
UPC
8 84682 00500 9
10 9 8 7 6 5 4 3 2 1
Made in the USA

BUILDING A SURVIVAL KIT – A Waterproof Folding Guide to the Key Components for Wilderness Survival

PATHFINDER OUTDOOR SURVIVAL GUIDE™

BUILDING A SURVIVAL KIT

A Waterproof Folding Guide to the Key Components for Wilderness Survival

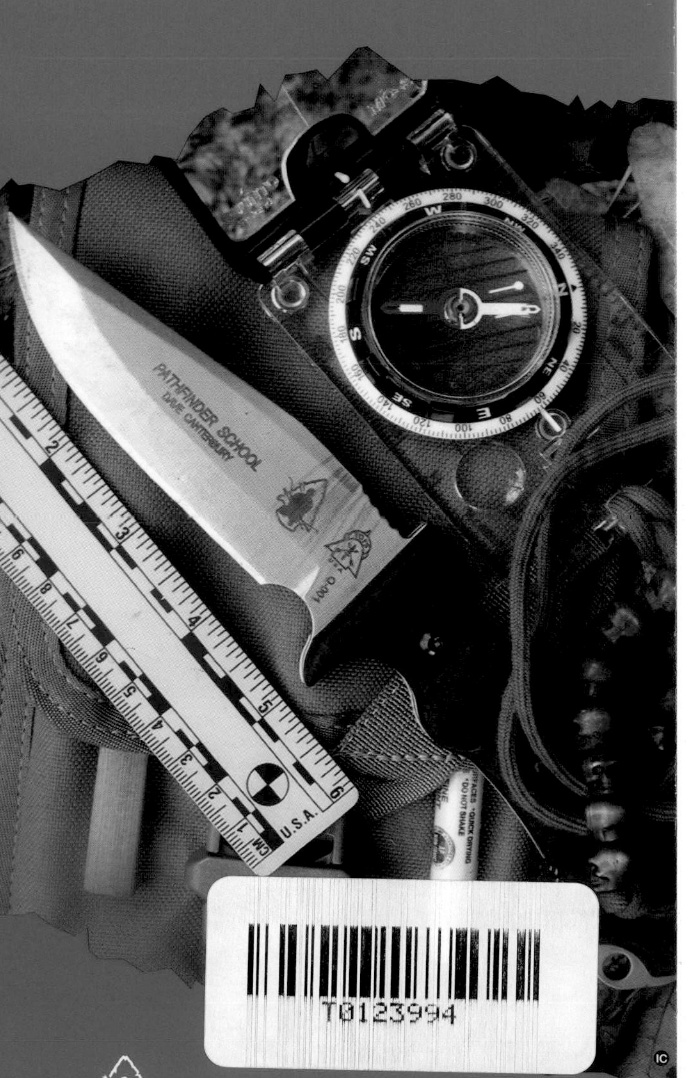

THE PATHFINDER SCHOOL
www.thepathfinderschoolllc.com

SURVIVAL KIT ESSENTIALS

Basis of Reasoning in Building an Emergency or Everyday Kit

Mental preparation and awareness play a key role in survival. Add a few basic tools and you have everything you need to survive in an emergency situation.

All of the tasks you need to accomplish in a wilderness emergency require energy. That means burning calories. Survival is about managing the energy you have, and knowing how to restore or replenish your strength while you wait for rescue or attempt to get yourself out of your situation. In all instances, weigh the trade-off of preserving hydration and energy versus the benefits of the task.

70% of your average caloric intake and hydration burns through normal daily activities – add stress and the need to expend energy to survive in the wilderness and it becomes essential to limit any extra exertion. You do this by carrying the essential kit basics.

With the items in your survival kit and some ingenuity, you should be able to beat a 72-hour scenario – the minimum amount of time you should prepare for. Remember, this is an "emergency" gear kit, so strive for the minimum. Your "add-ons" for other uses are up to you, but don't skip any of the basics.

Your kit essentials are the tools for tasks that would, in a survival situation, take the greatest amount of energy to perform without them.

The five most important tools are:

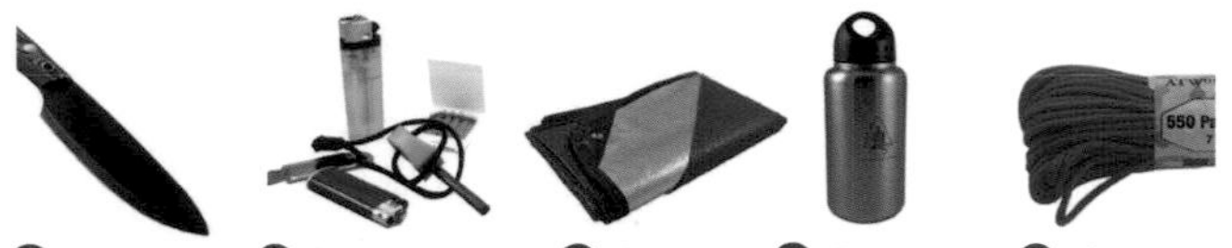

1. Cutting Tool (knife)
2. Combustion Source
3. Cover (shelter)
4. Container
5. Cordage

The five second most important tools are:

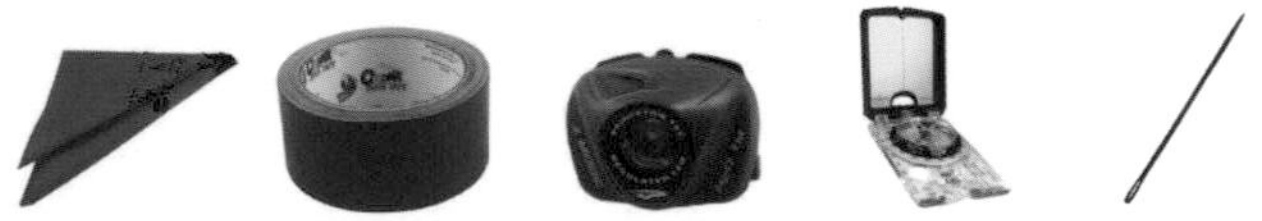

6. Cotton Bandana
7. Cargo Tape
8. Candling Device
9. Compass
10. Canvas Needle

Together, these items comprise the 10 C's of Survivability

Kit Basics

Have – and know how to use – the right equipment. Each individual (even children) should have their own survival kit with them. In the event that you get separated or swept downriver, each person may be facing their own survival emergency.

- Buy the best equipment you can afford.
- Don't carry unnecessary items.
- Have the five key components on your body – strap your knife to your body so if your boat tips, or you lose your pack, you have the basics to ensure your survivability with what remains.

Note: All gear for emergency use by children should be blaze orange if possible. Items that cannot be found in blaze orange should be wrapped in orange tape – either electrical or duct tape will do the job. Use common sense about knives and kids – teach them to safely handle a knife if you place one in their kits.

SURVIVAL KIT ESSENTIALS

Your Pack

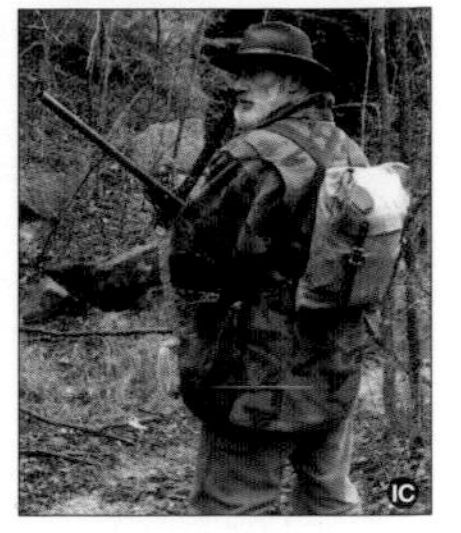

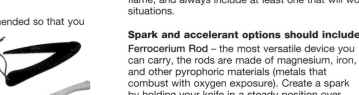

My focus is on functionality, a surplus pack will do the job but it must have the capacity to accommodate your survival kit basics plus any personal items. The larger the pack, the more you will clutter it with unnecessary items. It is always better to carry more knowledge in your head and fewer extras in your pack.

For pack construction, always look at these three factors:

Material – canvas or 500 dernier fabric at minimum, so it doesn't tear if you slide down a rock face.

Capacity – 35 to 70 liter capacity; the fewer pockets the better. Open bucket style packs are always the best option for easy access.

Closures – the quality of the zips, buckles and straps is vital. A pack won't do you any good if the closures break, or if you can't get it open without destroying it. Rough it up when you are testing it before buying.

1. CUTTING TOOL

If you have one thing, have a knife. It is your most valuable asset and you can do almost anything, except find water, with a good knife. A knife will help you build shelter, cut firewood, prepare food and in extreme situations, serve as a defensive tool.

Not all knives are created equally. Spend the money once on a good knife, so you never have to spend it again. Spend as you can afford, knowing that it is the one tool you may have to stake your life on, and make sure it meets these criteria:

Blade construction – full tang design. This means the entire knife is one solid piece of steel with handle bolted or pinned on. This becomes important if you need to baton your knife to cut fire wood. (Batoning means you will be striking down on your knife's spine with a piece of hard wood to use it as a wedge.) NOTE: don't use your knife unnecessarily to avoid dulling the blade. If wood can be broken, do that rather than using your knife.

Blade steel – high carbon steel like tool steel or 1095/01 or a spring steel like 5160. This gives you broad functionality as well as the ability to use it as a striker for true flint and steel fire starting in an emergency. Do not select a stainless steel blade or a coated blade, it will not work to make a friction fire, which you may need to do.

Blade spine – be sure the knife has a good 90 degree sharp spine and is non-coated. This is important for driving sparks generated by a Ferrocerium Rod. You should expect to spend anywhere from $100 to $350 for this single item, but its usefulness warrants the investment.

The Pathfinder Trade Knife and Pathfinder Knife PLSK1 are acceptable choices that cost under $100.

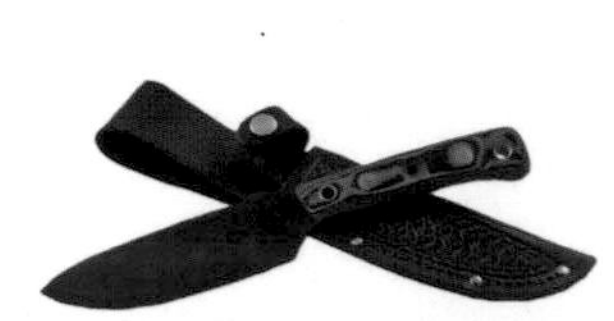

Pathfinder Trade Knife

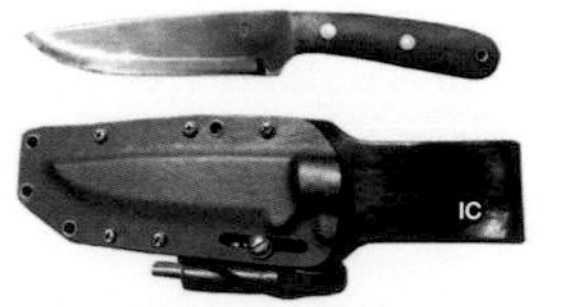

Pathfinder Knife PLSK1

1. CUTTING TOOL

In addition to construction, these elements affect functionality and should be considered as you choose your knife.

Blade length – the blade should be between 5" and 6". Too long and the blade will be useless for fine carving, too short and it will be no good for chopping, which is essential.

Blade grind and profile – the grind needs to be shallow enough for chopping, but steep enough to saw cut if needed. Too steep a grind will have a tendency to chip in cold weather or when chopping bone. This is a personal choice, but I prefer a Scandinavian type grind on a knife that looks similar to a large kitchen knife.

Blade thickness – a minimum of 3/16" is recommended so that you can use it for prying or batoning.

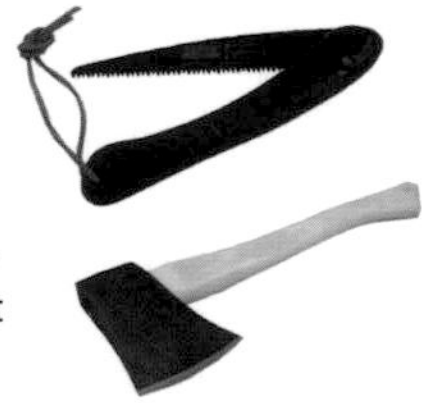

If you are dead set against carrying a fixed blade knife, carry a good 3" – 4" folding knife like the Opinel along with a good quality folding saw like the Bacho Laplander.

If you are in an area during heavy winter snow and with large coniferous trees, then your best cutting tool option may be an axe.

LAST RESOURCE

Make a Cutting Tool

While you can recreate the knife or cutting tool using natural materials, the energy you will have to expend is excessive.
If you have to fashion a blade/cutting tool, here's what to do:

1. Find a hard stone that flakes at the edges. The best stones are flint, chert (quartz), obsidian, basalt and quartzite.
2. Find a second heavier stone, suitable for holding in one hand, but shaped in such a way that you can control the striking point against your blank (to avoid destroying your blank, and more importantly, to avoid crushing your fingers on the hand that is holding the blank).
3. Chip at it with another hard rock, striking the edge at an angle to mimic the edge of primitive arrows. Don't hit downward at a 90 degree angle, this will make the flakes come off short and stubby and limit the tool's utility.

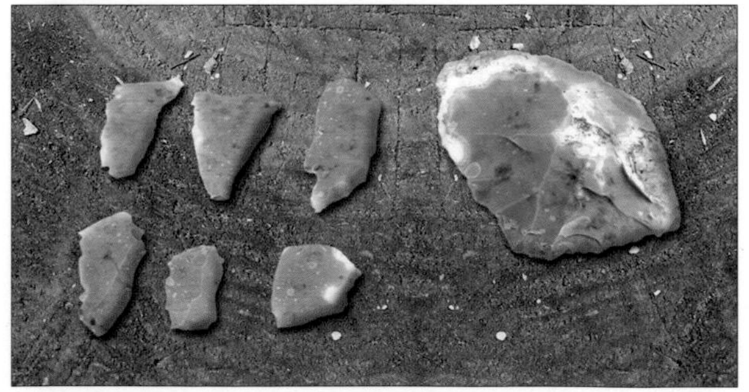

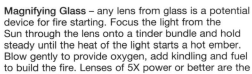

2. COMBUSTION DEVICE

It is not enough to just have a lighter to generate a flame; you must be able to make a fire in any weather or emergency condition. The romance of rubbing two sticks together – while absolutely imperative for you to know how to do – is a last resort since it burns too much energy and is not guaranteed.

Combustion devices must do more than create a spark. They need an accelerant that will light your tinder and hold a flame while you build the fire. There are a number of different options. Your combustion kit should include at least three different ways of making either ember or flame, and always include at least one that will work in extremely wet situations.

Spark and accelerant options should include:

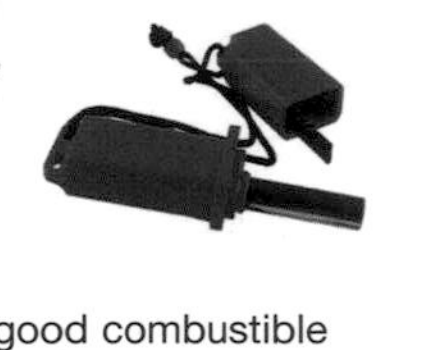

Ferrocerium Rod – the most versatile device you can carry, the rods are made of magnesium, iron, and other pyrophoric materials (metals that combust with oxygen exposure). Create a spark by holding your knife in a steady position over the target area and draw the ferrocerium rod toward you. The sparks from this device will be approximately 2000°F, which is enough to ignite good combustible tinder. Use in conjunction with Micro/Mini Inferno tinder. Spark from these rods is also great for use with char cloth or steel wool to produce an instant ember.

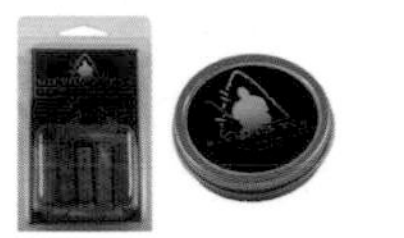

Chemical-based Accelerants – such as Mini Inferno or Micro Inferno are the best fire starting tinder available. They are individually packaged in tins that can be used to make char cloth or in smaller tubes that can be put into the Pathfinder Fire Striker.

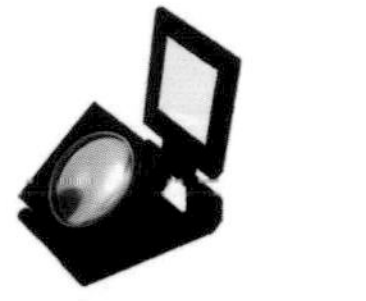

Magnifying Glass – any lens from glass is a potential device for fire starting. Focus the light from the Sun through the lens onto a tinder bundle and hold steady until the heat of the light starts a hot ember. Blow gently to provide oxygen, add kindling and fuel to build the fire. Lenses of 5X power or better are the most effective.

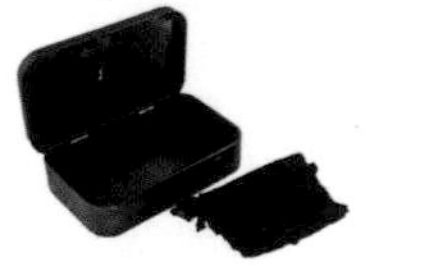

Char Cloth (100% cotton material) – combusts quickly and can be carried as a fire starter when you have to move locations. (See guide to *Shelter, Fire, Water* for instructions on how to make a char cloth).

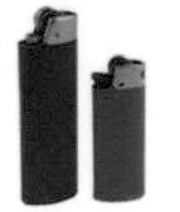

Lighters – In addition to your fire steel and magnifying glass, carry two BIC brand disposable lighters – **always orange for visibility** – wrapped separately in waterproof sandwich bags and taped by duct or electrical tape with a Micro or Mini Inferno in each.

The Ferrocerium Rod and Micro or Mini Inferno are the only products I would trust my life to. These sure-fire items will work even when soaked with water or at temperatures below freezing and they come packaged.

My personal kit contains a new lighter, 2 forms of chemical-based fire like Mini Inferno or Micro Inferno, a spare Ferrocerium Rod, steel wool, and a Fresnel lens wrapped in 100% cotton cloth for charring if needed. This is a well-rounded kit which costs very little and packs light and small. As with your knife, it is a good survival practice to keep a sure way to make fires attached to your body so it is readily available.

3. COVER

Shelter/cover is about creating a microclimate to protect you from elements that will affect with your body's core temperature and therefore your ability to function and think clearly.

It starts with clothing and being properly dressed for the conditions: In all circumstances, wear your clothes in layers to allow you to regulate your temperature by adding or removing pieces.

1. Carry or wear a hat in both hot and cold climates – in heat, a hat keeps you up to 15 degrees cooler than the surrounding environment. In cold, a hat will help restrict loss of heat through your head – a key conduction point on the body.

2. Wear "breathable" clothes to avoid sweating – wet clothes will cool your body quickly once you stop moving and will cause shivering, increasing caloric expenditure.

3. Remove wet clothing and get it dry - wet garments will increase your loss of body heat in cold climates. Alternately, use wet clothing to cool your body in hot environments.

Beyond that, you need a couple of items that will help to control your core temperature to avoid hypothermia (cold) or hyperthermia (heat). A couple of good re-usable emergency space blankets, a 55 gallon plastic drum liner and a wool blanket should suffice. Yes, I did say wool blanket, wool is the ONLY fabric that retains over 80% of its insulative value even when wet. You can also use these items to make shelters, shades, reflectors and signals.

Here are the shelter options that should be in your emergency kit:

1. **55 gallon drum liner** – (3 mil) or garbage bag (preferably ORANGE) suitable for use as a rain poncho, a sleeping bag or a lean-to style tent. This inexpensive and highly versatile shelter tool is lightweight, durable and reusable. You can move locations and carry it with you with minimal caloric expenditure. It takes up very little room in your kit, and has uses in both hot and cold climate situations.

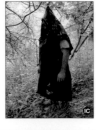

Drum liner uses include:
• Shelter construction • Rain gear • First aid
• Ground cloth • Signaling • Pack liner • Sleeping bag
• Water collection (water collected in a rainstorm doesn't need to be boiled before drinking) • Flotation device
• Dry storage (to protect important dry items like tinder)

2. **Space blanket** – Suitable for many of the same uses as the garbage bag, it should be carried in addition to the bag because of its light weight and versatility. A space blanket has one reflective side. In hot situations, put the reflective side out to deflect some of the heat of the sun, keeping you cooler. In cold weather the reflective side can be turned inward to hold radiant heat from your body to keep you warm. The reflective side can also be used for solar cooking and for signaling.

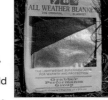

3. COVER

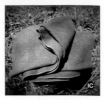

3. **Wool blanket** – is only likely to be carried if in a vehicle or backpacking situation. Wool is essential if you are outdoors in cold climates, but carrying it requires an expenditure of energy due to its weight, so consider the caloric trade-off against the potential risk when planning to include this in your kit. 100% wool is best and 80/20 is the minimum.

Regardless of the shelter tools in your kit, you should be familiar with basic shelter construction using the materials you have available. See the companion guide Shelter, Fire, Water for details on optional shelter construction.

LAST RESOURCE

If you find yourself without cover other than the clothes on your back, you will need to make choices to avoid the heat in warm climates (travel after the heat of the midday sun, stay out of the wind), or preserve body warmth in cold climates. Create layers of insulation between you and the elements; use leaves and other plant materials to provide additional protection from wind and cold.

4. CONTAINER

Containers are more important than most people think. Not only do they collect and carry water, they are useful for other purposes.

Any container must be able to withstand being placed in the fire – many stainless water bottles on the market will work and you need only remove the plastic lid and replace with a nesting cup to make char cloth, which gives you another option for the all-important fire. With this metal container you can: disinfect water by boiling, make medicinal herbal teas, or just warm your body core by using it as a hot water bottle. Use a highly polished container for an emergency signal mirror, to make char cloth and to cook small food items.

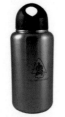

Stainless Steel Water Bottle   Drinking Cup/ Cooking Pot   Metal Canteen

LAST RESOURCE

If for some reason you have no metal container your immediate priority will be to carry water, this can be accomplished with your drum liner and your backpack. Containers can be fashioned from bamboo, as well as hollow logs. Boiling in these situations is tricky but can be accomplished by digging a hole, lining it with your other drum liner and heating rocks in the fire to stone-boil the water. Avoid using any rocks that are wet or near water for this operation as they may explode.

5. CORDAGE

Cordage is an important component of your kit. In the unfortunate event that you have to try to create a fire using the bow and drill method, durable cordage will be essential. Cordage uses include: shelter construction; bow drill fire string; net making, trapping & snares; self-rescue; fishing line; clothing and equipment repair; weapon construction; navigation/way-finding measuring devices.

Cordage is tough to re-create in large quantity so carrying it is always best. Cordages made with multiple plies can be broken down to finer fibers if needed. Polypropylene ropes are the least desirable type.

You should carry fishing bank line, which comes in 150# and 300# tests in large rolls. Being 3 ply, it can be separated to make fine cordage for fishing, sutures and so on. Make sure to purchase the tarred line if possible.

If you can't find the brand I recommend, make sure you have at least a 3 ply cord. I recommend carrying 100 ft. of lightweight Military Paracord 550#, which has 7 inner strands of nylon cord than can be unbundled to lengthen by that many times if needed. The original cord's strength is adequate in its raw form to suspend a hammock with a 220 lb. man, and will hold medium-sized game well, however paracord stretches a lot under tension and this must be considered during use.

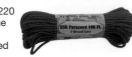

Cordage uses include:
• Shelter construction • Bow drill fire string • Fishing line
• Net making, trapping & snares • Self-rescue
• Clothing and equipment repair • First aid
• Weapon construction • Hygiene • Measuring

If you find yourself without cordage, you should know how to create it from the materials around you.

LAST RESOURCE

Make cordage: If you are without paracord, bank line or if you have lost your survival kit, then after a cutting device, you will need to make cordage to aid in making shelter.

The inner bark of hawthorne, hickory, poplar trees, stinging nettle and other fibrous plants are suitable for cordage materials (although this will not be strong cordage in comparison to fishing line or paracord). Prepare fiber by pounding, then clean the remaining fiber by hand. Peel out lengths of fiber, then "twist" or "braid" them to form long threads (keeping fiber wet while braiding will help with tightness and cordage integrity). Lengths are extended by adding in and twisting new pieces. Double and triple the first cordage lengths in a similar twining motion to create stronger rope.

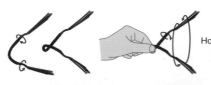

How to braid cordage from plant fibers

IN ADDITION TO THE FIRST FIVE, THERE ARE FIVE COMPONENTS I CONSIDER THE NEXT MOST IMPORTANT KIT ELEMENTS

6. BANDANA

I always carry 100% cotton bandanas that are at least 2' x 2'. If you have a choice of colors, choose orange so they can be used as signaling devices as well.

This is an indispensable item – I like having two – one on my head, and one (always blaze orange and large) in my pack. A military triangle bandage called "Drive on Rag" works well too, if you can find them.

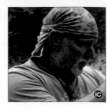

Bandana uses include:
• Make bindings and bandages for first aid • Wash rag for personal hygiene • To help cool your head and neck area on a warm day or insulate on a cool day • To gather edibles or transport other things • Be a first line water filter to remove large particles or turbidity (especially when used with charcoal from your fire) • To use part of one to make a char cloth for the next fire • To use as part of a sling for hurling rocks at potential game animals

7. CARGO TAPE

Cargo tape, or good old duct tape, is like a magic repair tool. It can manufacture nearly anything, repair most items and can even be used for first aid to bandage a wound or support a sprained ankle. Duct tape adhesive is also flammable so it will add to your fire arsenal. If the tape is orange it can be used to mark a trail or be used to leave a trace sign to indicate which way you went if you have to travel.

I recommend at least 20 ft. of 2 in. tape in a bright color such as orange or yellow, but if you can, carry an entire roll. Buy quality – you get what you pay for.

Cargo tape uses include:
• Lashing/cordage • Fire starter • Equipment repair
• First aid • Weapon construction • Container building
• Noise reduction • Arrow fletching • Improvised gear such as eye shades and sandals • Trail marking/blazing

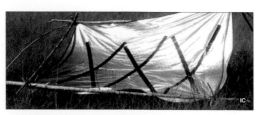

Use cargo tape on your space blanket to create a signal.

8. CANDLING DEVICE

Candling devices are lights, but not any light will do. You want a good waterproof headlamp that will also flash for signaling. Get a light that is at least 70 lumens, and preferably LED with multiple brightness settings. Different color lenses will make it more functional for night reading or blood tracking etc. If it has a flashing option, even better for signaling. Lights also offer peace of mind and help with the psychological factor of darkness until fire can be made. Avoid handheld flashlights because they limit your ability to use your hands when you are searching in the dark.

The Petzl Tak-Tikka is the one I have personally used and it has lasted for years. Try to use devices that take simple AA or AAA batteries, and carry a spare set taped with the purchase date written on them with your light. I carry my light in a small cord lock pouch with the spare batteries.

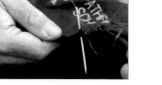

9. COMPASS

A compass is often overlooked with all the GPS and electronic devices, but when you can't reach a signal or your batteries have failed, the compass may be your only tool. Practice using it – they look simple, but in a high-stress situation, you want to know how to use it.

Your compass can be used to maintain a bearing to avoid lateral drift (walking in circles). A compass with a mirror can be used for signaling and for first aid to inspect areas like your face.

(NOTE: I have yet to find a magnifying glass built into a compass that will actually start a fire, so don't trust this compass function as part of your fire kit.)

As with other kit essentials, spend the money and buy the best compass you can afford with an adjustable declination and world needle. I recommend a Suunto MC-2 – it has a sighting mirror, several measuring devices and a magnifying glass.

10. CANVAS NEEDLE

A heavy stainless steel sailcloth needle or awl needle (for mending leather) can be used to repair fabric, or create bark containers or baskets. When magnetized, it serves as an emergency compass when floated on a leaf in water. It can also be used to dig out a splinter or stinger as well as remove debris from a wound, as a dart point, and in an extreme case, to suture an injury.

Be sure to buy a good quality stainless steel needle so it doesn't rust. The easiest ways to magnetize a needle are to place it on a magnet for several hours or use battery terminals to create an electric charge.

THE 10 C'S FOR SURVIVABILITY

The **10 C's** for Survivability:
Carry those items that would consume the most caloric energy to replace or substitute.

1. **Cutting Tool/Knife** – solid blade, suitable length for mixed uses, attached to your body
2. **Combustion Tool** – ideally at least three options – Micro or Mini Inferno (accelerant-based), Ferrocerium Rod, lighter, and magnifying glass)
3. **Cover/Shelter** – (reusable space blanket; two 55 gallon 3 mil drum liners, layers of clothes)
4. **Container** – (stainless steel 32 oz. minimum)
5. **Cordage** – 100' multi-ply (bank line/paracord)
6. **Cotton Bandana** – (100%) 2' x 2' minimum (ideally 3' x 3')
7. **Cargo Tape** – (duct tape - 2" wide)
8. **Candling Device** – (head lamp)
9. **Compass** – (with sighting mirror) and movable bezel ring
10. **Cloth/Canvas & Stainless Steel Sail Needle** – emergency first aid, mending clothes or shelter, improvised compass

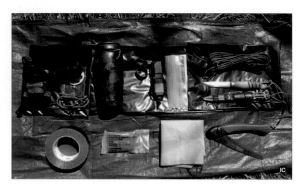

A LITTLE COMMON SENSE™

Study Your Environment

Your ability to find water, make fire, build a shelter, and find food will be greatly enhanced by familiarity with terrain, vegetation and climate.

Most survival concepts can be broken into three basic elements (The Pathfinder School "Rule of 3's"). If you can control three elements, you improve your survivability chances:

3 main killers to most lost or stranded people: hypothermia; hyperthermia; shock.

3 ways bodies gain or lose heat: radiation; conduction; convection.

3 basic needs for body function: rest; water; food.

Understanding these will allow you to maintain core body temperature and sustain yourself safely while you wait for rescue or attempt to find your way out of the situation.